# Title-
# "Art & Science Of Managing COVID-19"

## Author
### Dr Paridhi Shivde

MBBS, MD General Medicine

Professor in Department of General Medicine

Mahatma Gandhi Memorial (MGM) Medical College Indore, Madhya Pradesh, India

## Co-author
### Dr Neha Rai

MBBS, MD General Medicine (gold medal),

DM Neurology All India Institute of Medical Sciences (AIIMS) New Delhi (gold medal)

Consultant Neurologist Choithram Hospital and Research Centre Indore, Madhya Pradesh, India

# Preface

## Author
## Dr Paridhi Shivde

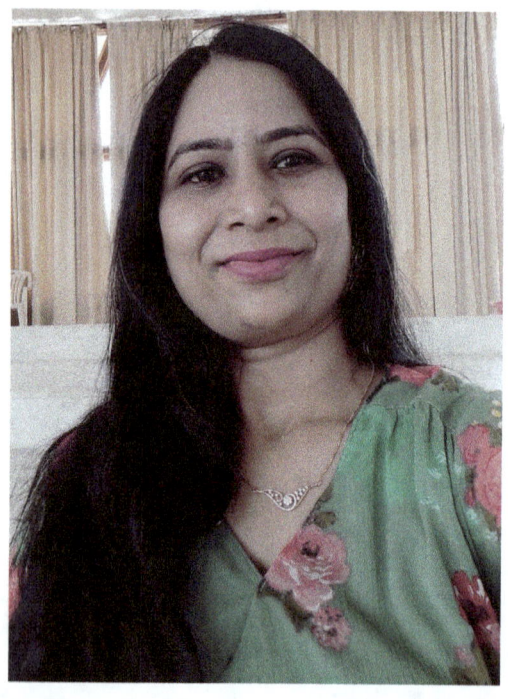

This book contains clinical presentations, complications, investigations, prevention and management of COVID-19.

It teaches the skill of identifying symptoms and signs, planning appropriate investigations, formulating a diagnosis and planning subsequent management. The book is written in a simple, specific, consolidated, comprehensive way and is less time consuming for treating clinicians and students.

The contents are very specific and in easy language.

# Preface

**Co-author**
**Dr Neha Rai**

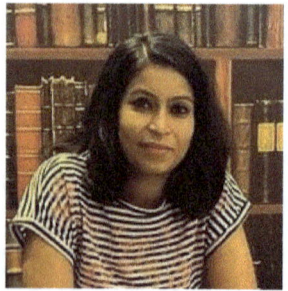

A concise and comprehensive description of clinical presentation, approach and management of COVID-19 is described in the book. The book can be studied in less time and is of value and help to practising clinicians and students.

# Acknowledgements

I, Professor Dr Paridhi Shivde thank my family members and well-wishers for their support and encouragement. A special thanks to my mother for her support. I thank my son Aviral for his constant support and invaluable encouragement.

I would also like to thank my Guru, International spiritual leader, humanitarian, ambassador of peace, Sri Sri Ravi Shankar (founder of 'Art of Living' organization) for his inspiration and teaching to serve society. His teachings have strengthened me and enabled me to face challenges in life. This book also has the intention of service.

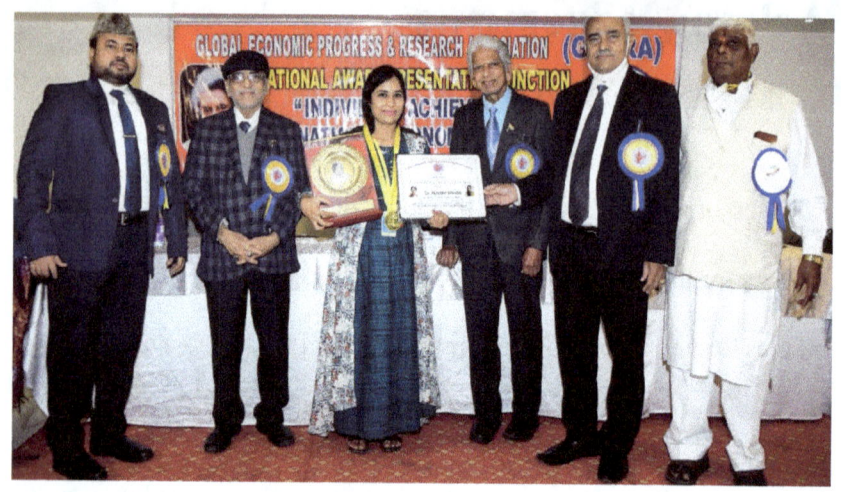

Dr Paridhi Shivde has received the prestigious Bharat Ratan Indira Gandhi gold medal award by Global Economic Progress & Research Association for her work in the medical and education field.

# CONTENTS

Chapter 1- Introduction to COVID-19

Chapter 2- Clinical presentation of COVID-19

Chapter 3 -Investigations in COVID-19

Chapter 4- Management of COVID-19

Chapter 5 -What does not work in COVID-19?

Chapter 6- Stages of COVID-19 disease

Chapter 7- Prevention of COVID-19 infection

Chapter 8- Cytokine storm

Chapter 9- COVID-19 in children

Chapter 10- COVID-19 vaccines

Chapter 11- Mucormycosis in COVID-19

# Chapter -1 Introduction to COVID-19

Coronavirus disease 2019 (COVID-19), the very contagious viral illness is caused by coronavirus.

COVID-19 disease has caused more than 3.8 million deaths worldwide.

The first cases of COVID-19 infection were first reported in Wuhan, China, in late December 2019.

The World Health Organization (WHO) declared it as a global pandemic on March 11, 2020.

Fig-1.1 Structure of COVID-19 virus

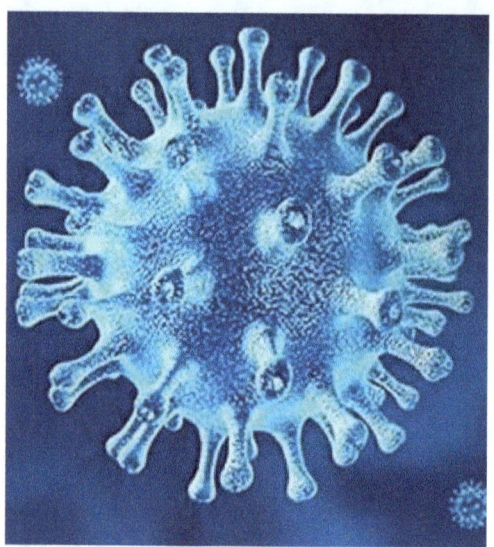

According to the WHO, as of December 11, 2021, five Variants of COVID-19 have been identified since the beginning of the pandemic:-

- Alpha
- Beta
- Gamma
- Delta
- Omicron

# Chapter-2 Clinical Presentation of COVID-19

## Clinical Presentation

Chief complaints-Fever, dyspnoea and cough are the main complaints.

• According to CDC(Centres for Disease Control and Prevention) in the US a report of 3,70,000 confirmed patient showed-

- Cough 50%
- fever 43%,
- malaise 36%
- Dyspnoea 29%
- sore throat 20%
- Diarrhoea 19%
- Nausea /vomiting 12%
- loss of a smell and taste, abdominal pain and rhinorrhoea less than 10%

❖ In some other studies loss of smell (anosmia) and dysgeusia (change in taste) were seen in 40% of patients. Initial symptoms of covid-19 disease- sore throat, running nose followed by cough, fever. Symptoms of viral illness are also present like fever, headache, myalgia, chills.

**Variations in clinical features**

- Vaccinated people have less severe symptoms and only mild symptoms like generalized weakness, headache and rhinorrhoea are present.
- Anosmia is found in a smaller number of patients who get infected with Omicron variant.
- Anosmia is more common in patients who get Delta variant infection.
- Symptoms vary from mild respiratory tract symptoms to severe pneumonia with acute respiratory distress syndrome to multi-organ dysfunction.

# Classification of COVID-19 diseases illness

**Asymptomatic or Pre-symptomatic Infection:**

People who have positive tests for COVID-19 infection using a reverse transcriptase-polymerase chain reaction test or rapid detection by antigen test but who have no symptoms that are consistent with COVID-19.

**Mild Illness:**

People who have any of the different presentations of COVID-19 (example-fever, cough, sore throat, malaise, headache, muscle pain, nausea, vomiting, diarrhoea, loss of taste and smell) but who do not have shortness of breath, dyspnoea, or abnormal chest imaging.

**Moderate Illness:**

Individuals who show evidence of lower respiratory disease during clinical assessment or imaging and who have an oxygen saturation (SpO2) equal to or more than 94% on room air at sea level.

**Severe Illness:**

People who have SpO2 less than 94%, 30 breaths/min, or lung infiltrates >50%.

**Critical Illness:**

People who have respiratory failure, septic shock, and/or multiple organ dysfunction.

*According to (World Health Organisation) WHO, 80% of COVID-19 infections are mild or asymptomatic, 15% are severe infections requiring oxygen and 5% are critical infections.*

**Happy hypoxemia**

Happy hypoxemia is the presentation of patients with extremely low blood oxygenation, but no sensation of dyspnoea.

# Clinical manifestations of covid-19

## Respiratory system involvement

- ❖ The respiratory system is the most common system involved in COVID-19 disease.

## Clinical picture

- o Viral pneumonia (most common presentation)
- o Fever
- o Cough
- o Dyspnoea occurs after 5-8 days of symptoms onset
- o Hypoxemia-pulse oximeter shows decreased oxygen saturation
- o Chest radiography shows bilateral infiltrates
- o Respiratory failure
- o Acute respiratory distress syndrome (ARDS)

- ❖ Dyspnoea increasing over time may be due to worsening pulmonary involvement, therefore in a patient attending outpatient department suspected of COVID-19 disease, Enquire for the presence of dyspnoea and check oxygen saturation. Also, advise the patient to check oxygen saturation by pulse oximeter twice a day at home.

# Cardiovascular system involvement

**Arrhythmias-**

- Most common arrhythmia found in COVID-19 disease is sinus tachycardia.
- Others arrhythmia are polymorphic or monomorphic ventricular tachycardia.
- Bradyarrhythmia like heart block is less commonly seen.

**Heart failure –**

- There is an increase in the incidence of acute heart failure in Covid-19 disease.
- In a small retrospective study of seriously ill patients in Wuhan, heart failure is seen in 49% of patients who died and 3% of patients who recovered.
- Analysis of 3080 consecutive patients with COVID-19 infection was done including a follow-up of 30 days. Out of the total patients, 77 patients (2.5%) who never had a history of cardiac illness were diagnosed with acute heart failure. The patients

suffering from or have a history of chronic heart failure (4.9%) developed acute decompensation after a COVID-19 infection.

**Myocardial injury** –

- Increased cardiac troponin level in 7 to 28% of patients.
- Myocardial infarction is also reported.
- Myocardial injury may be due to
  - stress cardiomyopathy
  - hypoxic injury
  - ischaemic injury (caused by cardiac microvascular damage or epicardial coronary artery disease)
  - systemic inflammatory response syndrome (cytokine storm)
- Cardiac troponin and natriuretic peptide (B-type natriuretic peptide -BNP and N-terminal pro-BNP -NT-proBNP) biomarkers are usually found elevated in hospitalized patients with Covid-19. These elevated markers are associated with an increased risk of mortality and are found in 7 to 36 per cent of patients. Cardiac troponin elevation is due to myocardial injury.
- In a study conducted in Germany, 100 patients with COVID-19 were enrolled. All the patients underwent cardiac magnetic

resonance imaging (MRI) 71 days after diagnosis. Cardiac involvement was found in 78% of patients and ongoing myocardial inflammation was found in 60% of patients.

- The increased production of inflammatory cytokines like interleukins(IL) IL-6, IL-10, and tumor necrosis factor Alpha (TNF-α) can lead to myocardial damage as well as stress-induced cardiomyopathy.

## Nervous system involvement

### Neurological Complications

- In half of the hospitalised patients some neurological complaints are present like headache, dizziness, myalgia, alteration of consciousness, disorders of the smell and taste, and fatigue.
- Encephalopathy is found in critically ill patients. MRI brain, EEG and CSF should be done.
- Stroke and seizures
    - Stroke is present in 1-6% of patients.
    - Ischaemic stroke is more common.
    - Haemorrhagic stroke and cerebral venous thrombosis (CVT) can also occur.
- Peripheral neuropathy is frequent in patients with COVID-19. It is mainly due to immune mechanisms or side effects of drugs used to treat COVID-19.

- Number of cases of Guillain-Barre syndrome is also reported. There was progressive ascending paraplegia, which evolved over one to four days.
- Rare cases of Acute disseminated Encephalomyelitis and meningoencephalitis are also seen.
- The mechanism may be a direct invasion of the virus in the nervous system. And, there is severe systemic inflammation due to cytokine release. Also, there is renin-angiotensin system dysfunction.

**Psychiatric manifestations**

Following psychiatric manifestations are reported in patients with COVID-19 disease-

- Anxiety
- Depression
- Insomnia
- Confusion and delirium

# Gastrointestinal system involvement

❖ Around 33% of patients with COVID-19 present with gastrointestinal symptoms rather than respiratory symptoms.

**The common symptoms are -**

- Nausea
- Diarrhoea
- Vomiting
- Decrease in appetite
- Abdominal pain

**Mechanism**

- Angiotensin-converting enzyme 2 (ACE2) receptor is largely expressed throughout the gastrointestinal tract. COVID-19 virus enters gastrointestinal cells via ACE2 receptors leading to direct damage to the gastrointestinal organs.

Following gastrointestinal complications are described in critically ill COVID-19 patients in various studies-

**Acute liver injury-**

- In around 60% of patients with COVID-19 disease there is an elevation in aspartate aminotransferase and alanine aminotransferase levels.

**Mesenteric ischemia –**

- The incidence of mesenteric ischemia is around 4 per cent in critically ill patients suffering from COVID-19.
- The patients usually present with severe acute abdominal pain, nausea, vomiting, and diarrhoea.
- Later on, hypotension, shock and even death are reported.

**Acute Cholecystitis**

**Acute pancreatitis**

## Nephrology system involvement

## Renal manifestations

- Acute kidney injury (AKI)
- Some studies suggest renal involvement in 6-7% of patients. According to kidney disease improving global outcome (KDIGO) criteria incidence of AKI in COVID-19 patients is 3–9%.
- CT scan of the kidneys demonstrated reduced density suggesting inflammation and oedema.

**Thromboembolic complications**

- The risk of venous thromboembolism (VTE) increases in 25 to 43% of patients in ICU often despite prophylactic anticoagulant therapy
- Pulmonary embolism
- Strokes were reported in less than 50 years of age of patients without risk factors
- Acute limb ischemia (ALI)-
  - Acute limb ischemia is found in severe cases of COVID-19 disease.
  - There is a decrease in perfusion to an extremity.
  - The patient presents with pain in the affected limb. The patient may develop paralysis of the limb.
  - The lower limb is more commonly affected.
  - On examination, there may be pallor of the limb and absent pulses.
  - Investigated by duplex ultrasound and CT angiography.
  - Treated with anticoagulants and surgical revascularization.

**Cutaneous manifestations**

There is a variety of skin manifestations reported in patients with COVID-19 disease.

Examples-

- Vesicular lesions
- Urticaria
- Maculopapular rash
- Pseudo-chilblains -erythematous papules on acral surfaces, especially on the hands and feet
- varicella-like eruptions
- Irritant and allergic contact dermatitis due to continuous use of masks and gloves
- necrotic vascular lesions
- Severe multisystem inflammatory syndrome with mucocutaneous involvement in children.

## Ocular manifestations

### Conjunctivitis

- Most common Ocular manifestations in patients with COVID-19 disease.
- Symptoms are redness in eyes, foreign body sensation, tearing, mucoid discharge, eyelid swelling, congestion and chemosis.
- Many patients with COVID-19 infection have conjunctivitis as the initial presentation.

### Episcleritis

### Uveitis

### Optic neuropathy

### Secondary infections- bacterial and fungal

# Chapter-3 Investigations in COVID-19

### For Covid 19 confirmation

**Real-time RTPCR** (reverse transcriptase-polymerase chain reaction) test

- Tested in the nasopharyngeal swab, oropharyngeal swab, sputum and bronchioalveolar lavage.
- It is a gold standard test for diagnosis of COVID-19 infection.

### Rapid detection by antigen test

- On May 20 it was issued emergency use authorisation (EAU) by FDA.
- Results come in 30 minutes

### Qualitative immunoglobulins (IgG /IgM) Antibody test

- FDA issued emergency use authorisation on September 20.

## CRP (C-reactive protein)

- CRP levels increases in severe inflammation
- According to study results, published in *open forum infectious disease,* increased CRP may be a predictive marker in determining, which patients with mild disease will progress to severe disease. So, it is the more specific marker to assess disease progression.
- It is cheaper, results come early and it should be serially repeated.
- In studies, CRP was found elevated in patients who died of Covid 19. So, it could be a promising biomarker for assessing disease lethality
- CRP levels of more than 100 mg per litre are significant. Normal is less than 8 mg/L
- Usually, increased D dimer is also associated with increased CRP levels.

## D-dimer

- D dimer— Predictor of thromboembolic condition.
- Increase in D dimer is associated with mortality.
- Normal D dimer level is less than 500 ng per ML. If more than 1000ng per ML it is considered significant.

## Lactate dehydrogenase (LDH)

- LDH— is associated with severe Covid disease
- Some studies also show increased mortality in patients with increased LDH but larger studies are needed to confirm this finding.
- LDH of more than 245 units per litre is considered abnormal. Normal is 110 to 210 units per litre

## Ferritin levels

- Hyper-ferritinaemia is associated with the inflammatory state.
- It is associated with the severity of disease and disease progression.
- More than 500 μg per litre is considered abnormal.

## Procalcitonin level

- It has great specificity in identifying sepsis and can be used in the diagnosis of bacterial infection.
- It may be associated with severe disease.

## Interleukins-6 (IL-6)

- Studies show increased levels of IL-6 seem to be associated with inflammatory response, respiratory failure, leading to mechanical ventilation and mortality in COVID-19 disease.

## Complete blood count (CBC)

- lymphopenia (83%) in hospitalised COVID-19 patients. It is associated with increased mortality
- Absolute lymphocyte counts less than 800/ microliter.

## Liver function test (LFT)

- Increase in liver enzymes

**Electrolytes**- serum sodium, potassium

**Blood sugar, HbA1c**

**Renal function test**-urea, creatinine

**Cardiac troponin and natriuretic peptide** (B-type natriuretic peptide -BNP and N-terminal pro-BNP -NT-proBNP) biomarkers

**Chest Radiographs-**

- Bilateral opacities or consolidation is the most common finding.

**High-resolution computed tomography (HRCT) chest-**

- American College of Radiology does not recommend a CT scan chest for screening or as a first-line test for diagnosis of COVID-19 disease because of variabilities of CT scan findings and findings may not be present in the first few days of illness.

**Electrocardiogram (ECG)**

**Echocardiography**

Fig-3.1 Chest radiograph showing bilateral consolidation in a patient with COVID-19

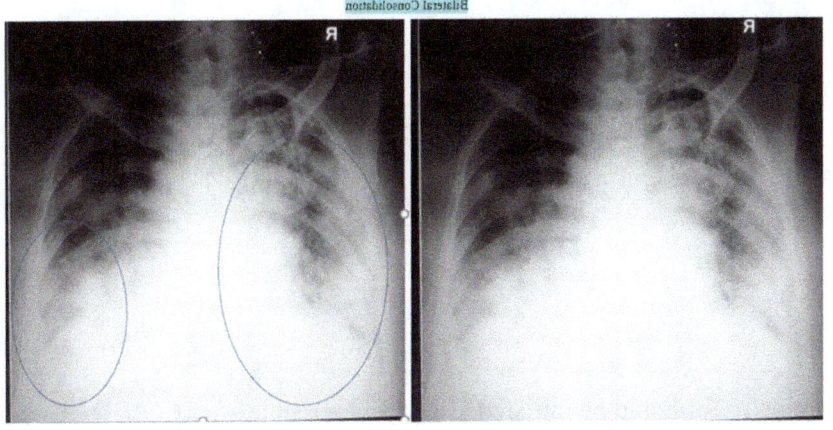

# Chapter-4 Management of Covid-19

## Treatment of Covid-19

### Antivirals

- *Any antiviral is most effective when used early in the course of the COVID-19 disease.*
- They should be initiated as early as possible after COVID-19 diagnosis and should be started within five days of onset of symptoms.
- Should use early in symptomatic patients with a lot of symptoms of viraemia including high-grade fever on days one and two, severe myalgia and prostrations.
- Decrease in viral load, duration of virus shedding and symptom improvement.

**Remdesivir**

- Remdesivir has got full approval from US FDA.
- Remdesivir acts by causing premature termination of viral RNA transcription.
- Eleven-year-old anti-viral drug and is largest evidence-based.
- Found effective against SARS (severe acute respiratory syndrome) virus and MERS (middle east respiratory syndrome) virus but was when tested against Ebola virus and Marburg virus, was found ineffective
- Many multinational randomised controlled trials on Remdesivir in severe COVID-19 infection, published in NEJM and LANCET, all show the same results. That is a shorter time to recovery in comparison to placebo (median 11 days as compared to 15 days, a patient getting well 3-4 days faster) but has no impact on mortality.
- Intravenous (I/V) use
- Single loading dose 200 mg and maintenance dose 100 mg daily

- Five days course is as effective as 10 days of treatment in hospitalised severe patients.
- According to the US FDA liver function test should be tested in all patients before starting Remdesivir and daily while receiving Remdesivir.

> Studies in the Journal of American Medical Association (JAMA) showed that in milder cases, Remdesivir may not be used or may not be needed.

> Therapeutic remdesivir treatment initiated 12 hours post-inoculation reduced clinical signs, virus replication in the lungs, and decreased the presence and severity of lung lesions.

> In the Solidarity trial, four drugs were evaluated and the results showed that remdesivir, hydroxychloroquine, lopinavir and interferon had little or no effect on hospitalized patients with COVID-19.

**Changes made in United States Food and Drug Administration (US FDA) over the course of time are-**

- In May 2020 US FDA limited the use of Remdesivir to patients with severe Covid-19 disease.

  At that time Remdesivir got emergency use authorisation (EAU) from FDA for the treatment of severe Covid-19 disease. Severe disease was considered when oxygen saturation is less than or equal to 94% in room air or there is a requirement for supplemental oxygen or requirement of mechanical ventilation

- But on 28 August 2020 FDA broadened emergency use authorisation for Remdesivir to include all hospitalised patients who have covid-19 disease irrespective of the severity of the disease.

- On 22nd October 2020 FDA fully approved Remdesivir for treatment of Covid-19 patients, 12 years of age or more and weighing 40 kg or more and requiring hospitalisation. Earlier Remdesivir was given only emergency use authorisation in hospitalised patients.

## Side effects of Remdesivir

- Hepato-toxicity —elevated hepatic enzymes
- Gastrointestinal — constipation, nausea, diarrhoea, vomiting, poor appetite
- Respiratory failure (Grien et al.NEJM)
- Cardiovascular— hypotension, atrial fibrillation, hypernatremia
- Renal— renal impairment, acute kidney injury
- Anaemia
- Other like Hyperglycaemia, Hypokalaemia

## Combination of Nirmatrelvir and Ritonavir

- An oral combination of Nirmatrelvir and ritonavir was issued an emergency use authorisation (EAU) by FDA for treatment of mild-to-moderate Covid-19 in patients (aged 12 years and older and weighing at least 40 kg) who have an increased risk of developing severe Covid-19 disease.
- It is given to patients attending the outpatient department.
- Dose – combination containing tablets nirmatrelvir (300 mg) and ritonavir (100) mg to be consumed together orally twice a day for 5 days.
- It should be started early within five days of symptom onset in a patient with Covid-19 disease.
- Not recommended in patients with severe renal disease and severe hepatic disease.
- Nirmatrelvir and ritonavir, both are protease inhibitors.
- Nirmatrelvir -It blocks the activity of the SARS-CoV-2-3CL protease, an enzyme which is essential for replication of Covid-19 virus

- Nirmatrelvir and ritonavir coadministration
- Ritonavir- It slows the metabolism of nirmatrelvir, so this main drug in the combination kit remains active in the body for longer period and maintains higher circulating concentrations.

❖ According to the Evaluation of Protease Inhibition for COVID-19 in High-Risk Patients (EPIC-HR) trial including 2246 unvaccinated adult outpatients with at least one risk factor for severe disease, nirmatrelvir and ritonavir combination, administered within three days of symptom onset, decreased the risk of hospitalization or death at 28 days by 89 per cent compared with placebo after Covid-19 diagnosis.

## Molnupiravir

- Molnupiravir got emergency use authorisation (EAU) from FDA to treat mild-to-moderate Covid-19 in adult outpatients aged 18 years or more who have increased risk for progression to severe disease, including hospitalization or death.
- Molnupiravir-It is a nucleoside analogue and inhibits replication of SARS-CoV-2.

- Dose- 800 mg tablets orally twice a day for five days.
- Contraindicated – in patients less than 18 years of age because it may affect bone and cartilage.
- Not recommended- in pregnancy and lactation

## FAVIPIRAVIR

- Experimental anti-viral drug
- Not FDA approved and has not got emergency use authorisation
- But available in many countries including India, Japan, Russia
- Works against a broad range of influenza viruses
- Used in mild to moderate Covid19 disease
- Side effects—Increased transaminases, diarrhoea, decreased white blood cell count, hyperuricaemia, increased triglyceride level
- Dose— Oral drug 1800 mg BD on day1 followed by 800 mg BD for 2-14 days
- A disadvantage is the high pill burden

## Antibody-based therapies (monoclonal antibodies and convalescent plasma)

### Convalescent plasma therapy

- FDA granted EUA (Emergency use authorisation) on August 23, 2020, for use of convalescent plasma in hospitalised patients with COVID-19. After this Mayo clinic which was coordinating FDA sponsored COVID-19 "expanded assess program" discontinued enrolment on 28 August 20.
- Eligible donors with high titres of antibodies are selected.
- Transfusion should be done to the patient early within three days of illness, as many patients who were planned for plasma develop their own antibodies for virus by around 10 days.
- **Adverse effects** like transfusion-transmitted infections example HIV, hepatitis B, hepatitis C, allergic reactions, anaphylactic reactions, transfusion-related acute lung injury, transfusion-associated circulatory overload and haemolytic reactions.

- Slight improvement in mortality was found in patients who received plasma in the Mayo group observational study.
- The National Institutes of Health (NIH), a part of the U.S. Department of Health and Human Services COVID-19 guidelines panel concluded on August 20 that there are insufficient data to either recommend for or against the use of convalescent plasma for treatment of COVID-19
- Cochrane review of convalescent plasma use in patients with COVID-19 (July 20) expressed uncertainty about the benefits of convalescent plasma in terms of mortality at hospital discharge, prolonging time to death or improving clinical symptoms at 7 to 28 days.
- Three randomized controlled trials did not show any mortality benefit example- Simonvich et al. and the PLACID trial. The PLACID trial enrolled patients with moderate COVID-19 pneumonia and randomized them to receive either placebo or convalescent plasma. Convalescent plasma did not decrease progression to severe disease or all-cause mortality at 28 days.

➢ A study published in 2021 found it did not prevent worsening of disease in high-risk patients when administered in the emergency department within the first week of their symptoms.

**Monoclonal antibodies**

The FDA issued an EUA (Emergency use authorisation) bamlanivimab-etesevimab on February 9, 2021. The EUA permits use in combination with or treatment of mild-to-moderate COVID-19 in adults and adolescents who are at high risk for progressing to severe COVID-19 and/or hospitalization.

The monoclonal antibodies are alternative options for COVID-19 specific therapy for symptomatic outpatients with risk for progression to severe disease.

**Following are the monoclonal antibodies, that have received an EUA(Emergency use authorisation) by FDA-**

- Sotrovimab
- Casirivimab-imdevimab
- Bamlanivimab-etesevimab
- Bebtelovimab

**Time of starting therapy-** as soon as possible after diagnosis and within seven days of symptom onset.

## Indication of monoclonal antibodies

- Used in patients with mild to moderate COVID-19 who do not require hospitalization or supplemental oxygen or who are at high risk of progression to severe disease.
- Patients who are at high risk of progression to severe disease are immunocompromising condition or immunosuppressive treatment, overweight (BMI 25–30), Chronic kidney disease, Pregnancy Sickle cell disease, Neurodevelopmental disorders (cerebral palsy or genetic or metabolic syndromes and severe congenital anomalies), Medical-related technological dependence (tracheostomy, gastrostomy, or positive pressure ventilation that is not related to COVID-19), Infants.

**Adverse Effects·** Hypersensitivity, including anaphylaxis, Rash, diarrhoea, nausea, dizziness, pruritis

## Doses of the monoclonal antibodies

- sotrovimab -500 mg as a single intravenous dose
- casirivimab-imdevimab -600-600 mg as a single intravenous or subcutaneous dose

- bamlanivimab-etesevimab – 700-1400 mg as a single intravenous dose
- bebtelovimab -175 mg as a single intravenous dose
  These drugs have also received EUA (Emergency use authorisation) for the treatment of non-severe COVID-19 in outpatients at risk for progression, and have been demonstrated in randomized trials to reduce the risk of COVID-19 associated hospitalization or death in such patients by approximately 70 to 85 percent compared with placebo.

- European Medicines Agency (EMA) had approved the use of the monoclonal antibody regdanvimab (40 mg/kg as a single IV dose, maximum 8000 mg) for outpatients with COVID-19 who have certain risk factors for severe disease and who do not require supplemental oxygen.

**Recent changes in guidelines for the USA due to increasing Omicron variant in Unites States of America**

- On January 24, 2022, FDA limits use of certain Monoclonal Antibodies to treat COVID-19 due to the Omicron Variant
- The two monoclonal antibody treatments – bamlanivimab-etesevimab and casirivimab-imdevimab are not found to be active against the omicron variant, which is circulating at a very high frequency (99% of Covid-90 patients) throughout the United States, these treatments are not authorized for use in any U.S. states, territories, and jurisdictions at this time.
- NIH (National Institute of Health, a part of the US Department of Health and Human Services) Covid-19 treatment guidelines panel also recently recommended against the use of these two monoclonal antibody combination treatment bamlanivimab-etesevimab and casirivimab-imdevimab because of their significantly reduced activity against the omicron variant and because real-time testing to identify rare, non-omicron variants is not routinely available.
- The COVID-19 Treatment Guidelines Panel (the Panel) recommends using sotrovimab 500 mg as a single intravenous (IV) infusion, administered as soon as possible and within 10

days of symptom onset, to treat nonhospitalized patients (aged ≥12 years and weighing ≥40 kg) with mild to moderate COVID-19 who are at high risk of clinical progression.

## STEROIDS

- In a meta-analysis of randomised clinical trials in JAMA shows that in critically ill patients with COVID-19, administration of systemic corticosteroids was associated with lower 28 days all-cause mortality in comparison to usual care or placebo.
- Large study "Recovery trial" showed that mortality rate was lower among patients who received dexamethasone in comparison to patients who received a standard care.
- But dexamethasone shows no benefit among patients who don't need oxygen or respiratory support.
- As we know Steroid is a most potent immunosuppressant and suppresses the patient's own immune system, it is said not to start steroids on day one, start it when the inflammatory response is more ($5^{th}$-$7^{th}$ day)
- **Chinese Thoracic Society** states that steroids should be used with caution in patients with hypoxaemia with COVID-19 and dose administration should be less than 0.5 mg per KG per day methylprednisolone or equivalent and for a shorter duration of

less than seven days. Short-term use is safe except for temporary hyperglycaemia.

- **NIH (National Institute of Health, a part of the US Department of Health and Human Services) treatment guidelines panel**
    - Panel recommends using dexamethasone 6 mg per day for up to 10 days or until hospital discharge in hospitalised patients who are on mechanical ventilation or requiring supplemental oxygen.
    - Panel recommends against using dexamethasone for the treatment of patients who do not require supplemental oxygen.
    - If dexamethasone is not available panel recommends alternatives such as prednisolone, methylprednisolone or hydrocortisone.
- **WHO Practical issues for the use of systemic corticosteroids in COVID-19 disease**
    - Medication route: orally or intravenously.

**Equivalent doses of steroids in COVID-19 for 7 to 10 days in patients requiring supplemental oxygen or mechanical ventilation are-**

- Dexamethasone- 6 mg once daily
- Methylprednisolone -32 mg (8 mg 6 hourly or 16 mg 12 hourly)
- Hydrocortisone –160 mg (50 mg 8 hourly or 100 mg 12 hourly)
- Prednisolone 40 mg once daily

## Anticoagulants

- Covid 19 patients frequently develop procoagulative state.
- The mechanism is poorly understood.
- It is caused by virus-induced endothelial dysfunction, cytokine storm and complement cascade activation.
- It is common to observe diffuse microvascular thrombi in multiple organs, mostly in pulmonary microvessels.
- High D dimer levels are associated with poor prognosis.

**National Institute of health US anti-thrombotic therapy in patients with COVID-19 May 20**

- Measure haematological and coagulation parameters example D dimer, prothrombin time, platelet count, fibrinogen in the hospitalised patients.
- All hospitalised patients with COVID-19 should receive the venous thromboembolism (VTE) prophylaxis. LMWH is preferred.
- Hospitalised patients with COVID-19 should not routinely be discharged on venous thromboembolism (VTE) prophylaxis.

## Immunomodulator- Interleukin 6 (IL-6) inhibitor (tocilizumab)

- Interleukin 6 receptor antagonist
- Tocilizumab is a FDA approved immunosuppressive drug for the treatment of active rheumatoid arthritis.
- Currently, FDA has not approved Tocilizumab for the treatment of COVID-19.
- On 24 June 2021, Tocilizumab is issued an EUA (Emergency use authorisation) for the treatment of hospitalized patients (2 years of age and older) who are receiving systemic corticosteroids and require supplemental oxygen, non-invasive or invasive mechanical ventilation, or extracorporeal membrane oxygenation (ECMO).
- Also used in the treatment of cytokine storm.
- Studies like EMACTA trial (September 20) show that Tocilizumab decreases the risk of mechanical ventilation or death in patients with COVID-19 pneumonia.
- ROCHE (healthcare Pharmaceuticals and Diagnostics company that operates worldwide) confirmed that Phase 3

COVACTA study (July 20) that Tocilizumab fail to meet the endpoints. The primary endpoint of improving clinical status in covid associated pneumonia and the Secondary endpoint of decreasing mortality.

- But ROCHE committed to continue the trial and also to study combination with antivirals.

- **The National Institute of health (NIH) US Panel** recommends using tocilizumab (single intravenous [IV] dose of tocilizumab 8 mg/kg actual body weight up to 800 mg) in combination with dexamethasone (6 mg daily for up to 10 days) in certain hospitalized patients who are exhibiting rapid respiratory decompensation due to COVID-19. These patients are:

    - Recently hospitalized patients (within the first 3 days of admission) who have been admitted to the intensive care unit within the prior 24 hours and who require invasive mechanical ventilation, non-invasive ventilation, or high-flow nasal cannula

(HFNC) oxygen (>0.4 FiO2/30 L/min of oxygen flow).
- Recently hospitalized patients (within the first 3 days of admission) not admitted to the ICU who have rapidly increasing oxygen needs and require non-invasive ventilation or high-flow nasal cannula oxygen and who have significantly increased markers of inflammation (CRP ≥75 mg/L)

- There is a risk of infections with the use of TOCILIZUMAB.
- Side effects are abnormal Liver Function Test (LFT), neutropenia, upper respiratory tract infections, nasopharyngitis, headache, increase in blood pressure, increase total cholesterol, dizziness, rash, gastritis and subcutaneous injection site reactions.

## Baricitinib

- Baricitinib is a Janus kinase (JAK) inhibitor that is approved for the treatment of rheumatoid arthritis.
- In November 2020 U.S. Food and Drug Administration (FDA) issued an emergency use authorization (EUA) for the drug baricitinib, in combination with remdesivir, for the treatment of COVID-19 in hospitalized patients (two years of age or older) who require supplemental oxygen, invasive mechanical ventilation or extracorporeal membrane oxygenation. Some data support the use of baricitinib alone without remdesivir.
- It has immunomodulatory effects.
- It is believed to have antiviral effects through interference with viral entry.
- It inhibits the intracellular signalling pathway of cytokines such as Interleukins(IL)- IL-2, IL-6, IL-10, interferon-$\gamma$, and granulocyte-macrophage colony-stimulating factor.

- It has been also shown to improve the lymphocyte count and prevent the entry of the virus into the cell.
- Tofacitinib is also a Janus kinase inhibitor, that can be used if baricitinib is not available.
- If tocilizumab is not available, Baricitinib can be an alternative in patients who are on mechanical ventilation or extracorporeal membrane oxygenation (ECMO).
- baricitinib is generally reserved for those who are within 96 hours of hospitalization or within 24 to 48 hours of initiation of ICU-level care, similar to the study population in the large trials.
- baricitinib is not usually administered in patients who have also received tocilizumab because both these drugs are not studied together and the safety of administering both the drugs together is uncertain.
- In a double-blind, randomized, placebo-controlled trial done in 1033 Covid-19 patients, coadministration of Baricitinib and remdesivir was superior to remdesivir alone in decreasing recovery time and speeding-up improvement in clinical status

among patients with Covid-19, among those receiving high-flow oxygen or noninvasive ventilation.

- Dose-4 mg orally once daily for up to 14 days.
- Not recommended- severe renal insufficiency
- Caution- in immunocompromised patients.
- Baricitinib or tocilizumab should only be given in combination with dexamethasone or another corticosteroid.

## Chronic Hepatitis B co-infection with Covid -19 disease-

- There is an increased risk of complications.
- As there is an increase in transaminases levels due to covid-19 infection and increased hepatotoxicity caused by covid-19 treatment, caution should be taken.

## HIV co-infection with Covid -19 disease-

- There is an increased risk of complications.
- Anti-retroviral drugs should not be stopped and in a newly diagnosed HIV infection patient, it should be started soon.

## Use of non-steroidal anti-inflammatory drugs (NSAIDs) in Covid -19 patients

- non-steroidal anti-inflammatory drugs (NSAIDS) should not be stopped and is to be given to a patient who has an indication for their use. US FDA, European medicines agency, World Health Organization (WHO) has got no evidence favouring that NSAIDS caused a clinical worsening in Covid - 19 patients.

## Use of angiotensin-converting enzyme inhibitors (ACE-inhibitor) and angiotensin receptor blocker (ARB) in Covid -19 patients

- No data supports that there is a more serious outcome in Covid -19 patients taking ACE inhibitors or ARBs, therefore these drugs should not be discontinued in patients who are on these medications.
- American Heart Association, the Heart Failure Society of America, and the American College of Cardiology all recommend that ACE inhibitors or ARBs should be continued in people who have an indication for these medications.

## NIH Covid-19 treatment panel guidelines-

**For patients with mild to moderate covid-19 disease, who do not require hospitalisation or supplementary oxygen**

**Preferred therapy**

- First preferred therapy – An oral combination of Nirmatrelvir and ritonavir
- Second preferred therapy- Remdesevir

**Alternative therapy**

for use only when neither of the preferred therapies is available, feasible to use or clinically appropriate, then either of these two drugs can be used as an alternative therapy-

- Bebtelovimab
- Molnupiravir

❖ The COVID-19 Treatment Guidelines Panel (the Panel) recommends against the use of dexamethasone or other corticosteroids for the treatment of COVID-19 for patients who do not require supplemental oxygen.

## For Patients Who Require Supplemental Oxygen

Recommendations

The Panel recommends using one of the following options for hospitalized patients who require supplemental oxygen:

- Remdesivir (example-for patients who require minimal supplemental oxygen)
- Dexamethasone plus remdesivir
- Dexamethasone- for patients on dexamethasone who have rapidly increasing oxygen needs and systemic inflammation, add a second immunomodulatory drug (example- tocilizumab or baricitinib)

## Patients Who Require Oxygen Through a High-Flow Device or Non-invasive Ventilation (NIV)

Recommendations

❖ The Panel recommends using one of the following options for hospitalized patients who require oxygen through a high-flow device or NIV-
  - Dexamethasone

- Dexamethasone plus remdesivir

❖ For patients who have rapidly increasing oxygen needs and have increased markers of inflammation, add either baricitinib or tocilizumab (drugs are listed alphabetically) to one of the options above.

❖ The Panel recommends using a prophylactic dose of heparin as venous thromboembolism (VTE) prophylaxis, unless a contraindication exists.

❖ The Panel recommends against the use of an intermediate dose (example-enoxaparin 1 mg/kg once daily) or a therapeutic dose of anticoagulation for venous thromboembolism (VTE) prophylaxis, except in a clinical trial.

**Patients Who Require Mechanical Ventilation or Extracorporeal Membrane Oxygenation (ECMO)**

Recommendations

- The Panel recommends using dexamethasone for hospitalized patients with COVID-19 who require mechanical ventilation or ECMO.

- The Panel recommends using dexamethasone plus tocilizumab for patients with COVID-19 who are within 24 hours of admission to the ICU.
- The Panel recommends using a prophylactic dose of heparin as venous thromboembolism VTE prophylaxis, unless a contraindication exists.

## Hydroxychloroquine

- It was initially started as a treatment for COVID-19 patients
- Studies show that Hydroxychloroquine have no impact on clinical outcome and mortality. Large studies like SOLIDARITY trial, RECOVERY trial, NIH (National Institute of health) US and NOVARTIS sponsored HCQS trial closed HCQS limb in the study and stopped it as the drug of trial and moved on with other drugs in trial.
- On July 19, World Health Organization (WHO) discontinues hydroxychloroquine and Lopinavir/ritonavir treatment arms for COVID-19 by accepting a recommendation from a SOLIDARITY international steering committee
- US FDA news release on June 15, 2020, in Coronavirus update says that FDA revokes (cancel) emergency use authorisation (EAU) for hydroxychloroquine in Covid 19.
- Not currently recommended for treatment of Covid 19.
- Side-effects of short duration Use of hydroxychloroquine
  - nausea, vomiting, diarrhoea, constipation, skin rash, QT interval prolongation, and ventricular arrhythmias.

# Chapter-5 What Does not work in Covid 19

## Antibiotics

- Antibiotics including, doxycycline, azithromycin have no role in treatment of COVID-19 disease except in secondary sepsis.
- According to a clinical infectious disease article, in the second or third week of severe hospitalised Covid disease, patients get secondary bacterial infections. But if more and early use of Antibiotics is done there will be
- pan-resistant infections

## Hydroxychloroquine

- Studies show that Hydroxychloroquine have no impact on clinical outcome and mortality.
- US FDA news release on June 15, 2020, in Coronavirus update says that FDA revokes (cancel) emergency use authorisation (EAU) for hydroxychloroquine in Covid 19.

### Oseltamivir (Tamiflu)

- It is approved for the treatment of influenza A and B. Study in Wuhan reported no positive outcomes in COVID-19. Several trials were still evaluating it in treating Coronavirus infections.

### Ivermectin

- Australian government has issued advice on inappropriate use of ivermectin for COVID-19 and stated that there is currently not enough evidence to show that Ivermectin is safe or effective to prevent or treat Covid 19.
- Chaccour et al also raise their concern regarding ivermectin associated neurotoxicity, particularly in patients with hyper-inflammatory states. Finally, evidence suggests that Ivermectin plasma levels with meaningful activity against COVID-19 would not be achieved without a potentially toxic increase in Ivermectin doses in humans.
- NIH (National Institute of health) US COVID-19 treatment guidelines panel recommend against the use of ivermectin for the treatment of COVID-19

- FDA issued a warning in April 20 that Ivermectin should not be used to treat COVID-19 in humans
- Side-effects of ivermectin
  - Neurotoxicity is the main concern.
  - Serious neurological side effects like dizziness, somnolence, vertigo, tremors, headache, vomiting, seizures, ataxia, disorientation, confusional state, coma.
  - Other side effects like fever, itching, skin rash, joint or muscle pain tachycardia.

### Vitamin C, vitamin D and Zinc

NIH (National Institute of health) US COVID-19 treatment guideline panel states *"there is insufficient data to recommend either for or against for use of vitamin C, vitamin D and Zinc"*

# Chapter-6 Stages of COVID-19 disease

## Stage I –

- early infection
- the first week of illness
- there is an increase in viral replication
- it is known as the viral responsive phase
- anti-viral drugs are effective in this stage
- plasma therapy conversion plasma therapy if indicated, it should be given in the first week of the illness

## Stage II

- pulmonary phase
- host inflammatory gets started leading to inflammation
- the second week of illness
- steroids and immunomodulators are used, if they are indicated

## Stage III

- inflammation increases
- hyper-inflammatory phase

*"Even if a patient starts stable, a patient can worsen from 7 to 10 days of illness due to the host inflammatory response phase"*

Figure-6.1 Preferred treatment in different stages of COVID-19 disease

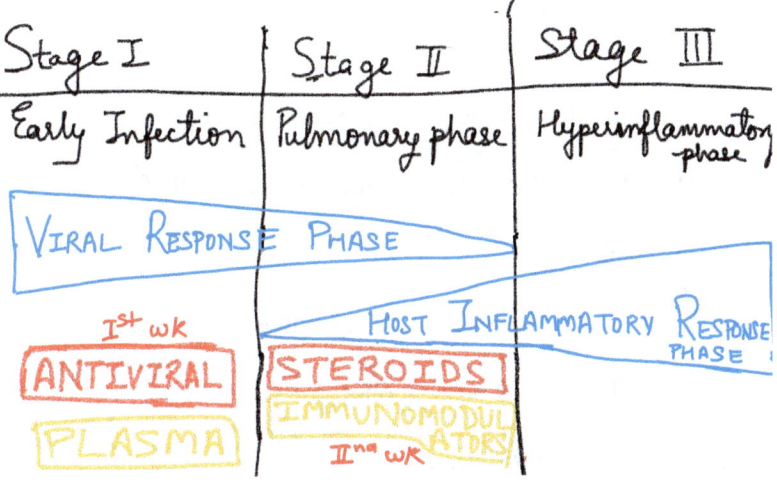

## Chapter-7 Prevention of COVID-19 infection

In the following ways, we can prevent COVID-19 infection-

- Get your Vaccination done as early as possible.
- Wear a mask on your face, especially in crowded areas.
- The mask should cover your nose and mouth. If you have not worn a mask, cover your mouth and nose with a tissue when you cough or sneeze, or use the inside of your elbow and do not spit.
- Wash your hands with soap and water for at least 20 seconds. You should not forget to wash your hands before eating or preparing food, before touching your face and after leaving a public place.
- When soap and water are not available, use a hand sanitiser containing at least 60% alcohol.
- Stay 6 feet away from others.
- Avoid places that are poorly ventilated and crowded.

# Pre-Exposure Prophylaxis- Monoclonal Antibodies

There are no clinical trial efficacy data on preventing symptomatic COVID-19 disease with the tixagevimab 300 mg plus cilgavimab 300 mg dose.

Factoring in the limitations outlined above:

**The NIH (National Institute of health) US Panel** recommends using tixagevimab 300 mg plus cilgavimab 300 mg administered as 2 consecutive 3 mL intramuscular injections as COVID-19 Pre-exposure prophylaxis for a person aged ≥12 years and weighing ≥40 kg who do not have COVID-19 infection, who have not been recently exposed to an individual with COVID-19 infection, who have not previously received this regimen, AND who:

- Are moderately to severely immunocompromised and may have inadequate immune response to COVID-19 vaccination, or
- Are not able to be fully vaccinated with any available COVID-19 vaccines due to a history of severe adverse reaction to a COVID-19 vaccine or any of its components.
- For patients who have previously received a dose of tixagevimab 150 mg plus cilgavimab 150 mg, the FDA EUA

states that a second dose of tixagevimab 150 mg plus cilgavimab 150 mg should be given as soon as possible.
- Tixagevimab plus cilgavimab is not a substitute for COVID-19 vaccination and should not be used in unvaccinated individuals for whom COVID-19 vaccination is recommended and who are anticipated to have an adequate response.
- Individuals who qualify as having moderate to severe immunocompromising conditions under the FDA EUA for tixagevimab plus cilgavimab are those who:
  - Are receiving active treatment for solid tumors and hematologic malignancies.
  - Received a solid organ transplant and are receiving immunosuppressive therapy.
  - Received chimeric antigen receptor T cell therapy or a hematopoietic stem cell transplant (within 2 years of transplantation or receiving immunosuppression therapy).
  - Have a moderate or severe primary immunodeficiency (e.g., DiGeorge syndrome, Wiskott-Aldrich syndrome).

- Have advanced or untreated HIV infection (defined as people with HIV and CD4 T lymphocyte counts

## Post-Exposure Prophylaxis

- The NIH (National Institute of health) US Panel recommends against the use of bamlanivimab plus etesevimab and casirivimab plus imdevimab for post-exposure prophylaxis (PEP), as the Omicron variant, which is not susceptible to these agents, is currently the predominant variant circulating in the United States.
- The Panel recommends against the use of hydroxychloroquine for COVID-19 Post-Exposure Prophylaxis
- The Panel recommends against the use of other drugs for COVID-19 Post-Exposure Prophylaxis, except in a clinical trial.

# Chapter-8 Cytokine storm

**Cytokine storm** is an umbrella term for a group of hyperactive immune responses triggered by-

- Infections
- Complication of autoimmune or autoinflammatory diseases
- Cancer or therapy of cancer
- Most common infections causing it are viral infections like Epstein bar virus, herpes simplex virus, influenza virus, 2009 H1N1, cytomegalovirus virus and now this nasty Covid 19 infection.
- Lymphocytes kill viral infected cells and interaction between them leads to an increase in pro-inflammatory cytokines like Interleukins (IL)-IL6, IL12, IL-1 beta, Tumour necrosis factor alpha (TNF alpha)
- Result is multiorgan failure.
- Most prominent organ involvement is of the lung. Patients may present with acute respiratory distress syndrome (ARDS).

- Others like kidney (acute kidney injury), liver, central nervous system and heart are also affected
- DIC and thrombocytopenia are also reported
- A hallmark of a cytokine storm is persistent fever and non-specific constitutional symptoms (weight loss, joint and muscle pain, fatigue, headache). Progressive widespread systemic inflammation leads to a loss of vascular tone that is manifested as a drop in blood pressure, vasodilatory shock, and progressive organ failure. Respiratory failure is the most prominent feature.

## Diagnosis

Cytokine storm is very difficult to diagnose and no single parameter is diagnostic.

Progressive hypoxemia

+

1 of the following (hypotension by 10 mm of mercury or fever more than or equal to 38.3 degrees Celsius

and

IL 6 more than 80 picogram per ml

or

All of the following (D-dimer more than one microgram per ml, CRP -C-reactive protein level more than 10 mg, ferritin more than 750 nanograms per ml)

## Management of cytokine storm

**Investigations** pointing to the cytokine storm are increased ferritin, CRP (C-reactive protein) , d-dimer, Interleukins -IL6 and Lactate dehydrogenase- LDH.

**Treated by**

- Glucocorticoid (immunosuppressants) but the side-effect is secondary infections and worsening of diabetes.
- Tocilizumab- IL6 receptor antagonist
- Anakirna IL1 receptor antagonist. According to NIH treatment guidelines, there is insufficient data in favour or against its use in Covid 19.

# Chapter-9 COVID-19 in Children

## Features of COVID-19 disease in children

- Usually, children have asymptomatic, mild, or moderate COVID-19 disease and recovery occur within one to two weeks of the onset of symptoms.
- But severe and sometimes fatal COVID-19 disease is found in some children.
- Multisystem inflammatory syndrome in children (MIS-C) is inflammation of multiple systems and organs like the heart, lungs, kidneys, brain, skin, eyes, or gastrointestinal system.
- The clinical features of Multisystem inflammatory syndrome in children resemble the features of Kawasaki disease.
- The most common age of involvement is 6 to 12 years of age.

# Treatment of COVID-19 in children

## Remdesivir

- Remdesivir is the only drug approved by the US Food and Drug Administration (FDA) for the treatment of COVID-19 in hospitalized paediatric patients (aged ≥12 years and weighing ≥40 kg).
- Remdesivir is also issued an FDA Emergency Use Authorization (EUA) for the treatment of COVID-19 in hospitalized paediatric patients weighing 3.5 kg to <40 kg or aged <12 years and weighing ≥3.5 kg.

## Baricitinib

FDA has also issued an Emergency Use Authorization (EUA) for the use of baricitinib in combination with remdesivir in hospitalized children aged ≥2 years with COVID-19 who require supplemental oxygen, mechanical ventilation, or extracorporeal membrane oxygenation (ECMO)

# Chapter-10 COVID-19 Vaccines

- There are many COVID-19 vaccines validated for use by WHO (given Emergency Use Listing).
- The first mass vaccination programme started in early December 2020.
- COVID-19 vaccines protect everyone ages 5 years and older from getting infected and severely ill, and
- COVID-19 vaccines also prevent infection by Delta or other variants.
- Side effects of vaccination are injection site pain, fever, fatigue, headache, myalgia. Anaphylaxis and myocarditis are side effects.

❖ COVID-19 vaccines are effective at preventing infection, serious illness, and death.

❖ Since vaccines are not 100% effective at preventing infection, some people who are fully vaccinated will still get COVID-19.

- ❖ The first vaccine to gain full FDA approval was mRNA-COVID-19 vaccine in August 2021. The FDA also has granted EUAs for 2 other SARS CoV-2 vaccines since December 2020. The mRNA-1273 and a viral vector vaccine – Ad26.COV2. S.

*"COVID-19 vaccines remarkably reduce the risk of hospitalization, serious illness and death, if a person gets COVID-19 disease."*

# Chapter-11 Mucormycosis in COVID-19

- ❖ According to the Lancet January 2022, the Year 2021 has also witnessed an unprecedented nested epidemic of COVID-19-associated mucormycosis that predominantly affected the Indian subcontinent. By July 15, 2021, India had recorded 45 374 cases of COVID-19-associated mucormycosis.
- ❖ According to the Centers for Disease Control and Prevention (CDC), USA On July 15, 2021, the Secretary of Health of Honduras (SHH), Central America was notified of an unexpected number of mucormycosis cases among COVID-19 patients.

## Mucormycosis

- Mucormycosis is an infectious disease caused by a fungus of class zygomycetes and the order of Mucorales
- Sometimes known as" black fungus".

- These organisms are ubiquitous and can be found on decaying vegetation and in the soil.
- These fungi grow rapidly and release large numbers of spores that can become airborne.
- These infections are usually acquired when spores are inhaled or, less commonly, enter the body through a cut in the skin.
- Mucormycosis is an aggressive, life-threatening infection that occurs in people whose immune system doesn't function well (immune-compromised) including people with uncontrolled diabetes mellitus.

## Causes of Mucormycosis in COVID-19

**Extensive use of the following drugs lead to the development of mucormycosis in COVID-19-**

- Steroids (in higher unrecommended doses)
- Immunomodulator- Interleukin 6 (IL-6) inhibitor (tocilizumab)
- Monoclonal antibodies (example-bamlanivimab-etesevimab
- Broad-spectrum antibiotics

- Steroids and Interleukin 6 (IL-6) inhibitor (tocilizumab) are immuno suppressants and increase the risk of secondary infections including mucormycosis.
- Monoclonal antibodies can block or reduce immune cells and cytokines, and can lead to increased risk of infection.

**Risk factors for Mucormycosis in COVID-19 are-**

diabetes mellitus, especially with diabetic ketoacidosis, treatment with Glucocorticoids, haematological malignancy, haemopoietic cell transplantation, organ transplantation, treatment with deferoxamine, iron overload and AIDS.

**Onset of Mucormycosis in COVID-19**

*"Cases of Mucormycosis are diagnosed several days to a couple of weeks after COVID-19 infection."*

## Clinical Presentation of Mucormycosis

Fig-11.1 Pathogenesis of Mucormycosis

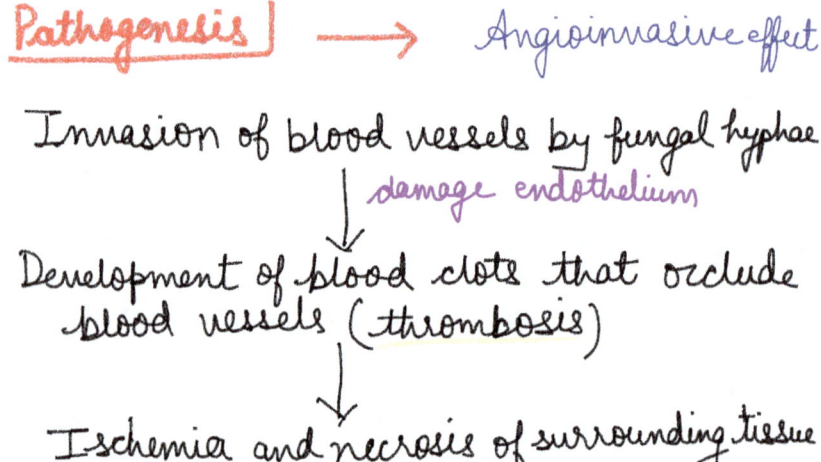

## Clinical features

1) Rhino- orbital-cerebral mucormycosis

2) Pulmonary mucormycosis

3) Gastrointestinal mucormycosis

4) Cutaneous mucormycosis

# Rhino-orbital-cerebral mucormycosis

## Sinus Involvement –

- Acute sinusitis with fever, nasal congestion, purulent nasal discharge, headache.
- Spread to cavernous sinus results in cranial nerve palsies (2nd to 6th cranial nerves), thrombosis of sinus and involvement of carotid artery.
- From sinuses infection spreads to palate, orbit and brain

## Palate involvement

- Necrosis and palatal eschars.
- Perinasal swelling, erythema and cyanosis of facial skin overlying in involved sinuses and /or orbit.
- A black eschar that results from necrosis of tissue visible in the nasal mucosa, palate or skin overlying orbit.

## Orbital involvement

- It is seen in moderately advanced disease
- Periorbital swelling, pain in the eye
- Double vision
- Loss of vision or blindness

- Dropping of eyelid or proptosis
- Facial numbness and swelling on the same side

**Cerebral involvement**

- Vascular invasion – brain ischemia or infarction including the cerebrum, cerebellum and brainstem.
- Diffuse vasculitis weakens blood vessels leading to the formation of aneurysms. Rupture of aneurysmal blood vessels causes subarachnoid, subdural or intracerebral haemorrhages.

**Pulmonary mucormycosis –**

- Pneumonia with infarction and necrosis
- It is rapidly progressive.

**Gastrointestinal mucormycosis –**

- Abdominal pain, haematemesis
- Necrotic ulcers in the stomach, oesophagus or intestine lead to perforation and peritonitis.

**Cutaneous mucormycosis-**

- Single or indurated areas of cellulitis leading to necrotic lesions.
- There may also be abscesses, skin swelling and necrosis.

Fig-11.2 Necrosis in the palate and palatal eschars in a patient with mucormycosis

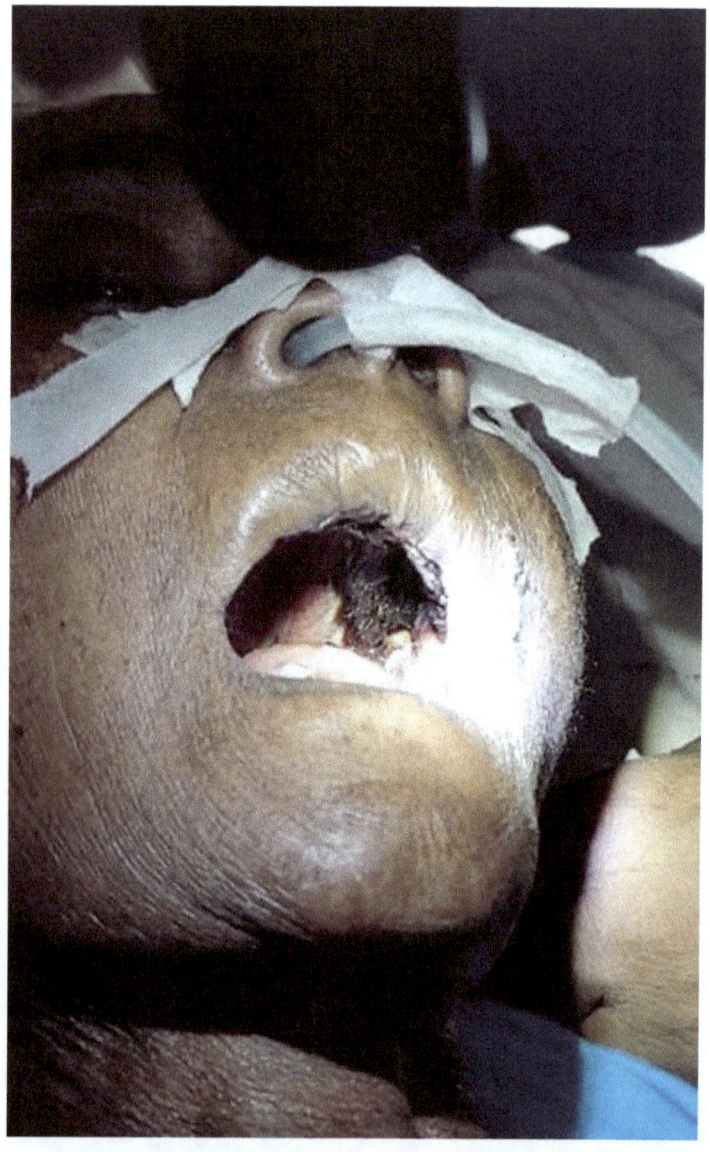

## Investigations

- Analysis of biological specimens from affecred sites is essential for diagnosis.
- Get tissue biopsies for histopathology and culture of the organism.
- Biopsy of necrotic tissue are taken from involved sites like nasal, palatine, lung, cutaneous, gastrointestinal , or abscess wall sites.
- Cultures, usually shows no growth.
- Despite angioinvasive nature of the organism, blood cultures are usually negative
- histopathologic identification of an organism with a structure typical of Mucorales may provide the only evidence of V
- Vascular invasion and necrosis are the typical consequences. There is neutrophil infiltration, vessel invasion, and tissue infarction. There may be a granulomatous reaction.

- Endoscopic evaluation of sinuses to diagnose tissue necrosis and also to take a biopsy.

## Other routine Investigation

- **Complete blood count** – decrease in neutrophils
- **Blood sugar** – fasting blood sugar, post-meal blood sugar, HbA1c
- **Serum Electrolytes**
- **Arterial blood gas analysis** to detect acidosis
- **Iron studies** to detect iron overload

    Increase ferritin, decrease total iron-binding capacity

- **Cerebrospinal fluid (CSF)**– increase proteins
- **Head and facial CT scans**
    - should be used as the initial investigation of rhinocerebral infections.
    - show sinusitis of the ethmoid and sphenoid sinuses, as well as orbital and intracranial extension.
    - bony erosion may occur and the infection may spread into the brain or orbits.

- thromboses of the cavernous sinus or internal carotid artery.
- infarct in different areas of the brain.
- CT scan head is more sensitive than MRI to detect bony erosion.

- **Magnetic resonance imaging (MRI) of facial sinuses and brain**
    - It is superior to a CT scan in assessing the degree of tissue invasion and need for ongoing surgery

- **Investigation of pulmonary mucormycosis**

    **Non-enhanced high-resolution CT scan of chest** is the imaging modality of choice.
    - Common findings - are pleural effusion, nodules, consolidation, and ground-glass opacities.
    - Reverse Halo sign (a nodule with central ground-glass opacity and a ring of peripheral consolidation) firmly suggest pulmonary mucormycosis and is rarely seen in invasive aspergillosis.

- Halo sign (a nodule surrounded by ground-glass opacity) suggest a lung infarct surrounded by alveolar haemorrhage.

o **Gastrointestinal disease**

- Abdominal CT scans may show a mass associated with the GI tract.
- Esophagogastroduodenoscopy (EGD) may show areas of tissue necrosis amenable to biopsy.

## Treatment of Mucormycosis

**Treatment of rhinocerebral mucormycosis includes the following:**

1) **Reversing underlying immunocompromised states**
2) **Administering systemic antifungals**
3) **Performing urgent surgical debridement**

o Antifungal therapy alone and surgical therapy by itself may be ineffective.

- Correcting hypoxia, acidosis, hyperglycaemia, and electrolyte abnormalities are necessary for successful management of this condition
- Discontinuation or maximally reducing immunosuppressive therapy like steroids, tocilizumab and monoclonal antibodies should be done.

## Surgical treatment

- Aggressive surgical debridement of involved tissues should be considered as soon as the diagnosis of any form of mucormycosis is suspected.
- Surgical intervention with removal of necrotic tissue and debulking infection has been associated with improved survival in clinical reviews of rhinocerebral and pulmonary infection.
- In the case of rhino-cerebral infection, debridement to remove all necrotic tissue can often be disfiguring, due to the removal of the palate, nasal cartilage, or the orbit.
- Orbital exenteration is needed in severe orbital involvement.
- Multiple surgeries may be needed.

- Endoscopic debridement with limited tissue removal can be tried.
- Early pulmonary infection can be treated with lobectomies.

**Medical treatment**

**Two main classes of antifungal medications used to treat mucormycosis are-**

1) polyenes (amphotericin formulations)

2) triazoles (isavuconazole and posaconazole).

**FDA approved drugs for the primary therapy**

1) Amphotericin B

2) Isavuconazole

**Initial therapy**

Intravenous (IV) amphotericin B (a lipid formulation) is the drug of choice for initial therapy.

**Step-down therapy**

Posaconazole or isavuconazole is used as step-down therapy for patients who have responded to amphotericin B.

## Salvage therapy

Posaconazole or isavuconazole can also be used as salvage therapy for patients who don't respond to or cannot tolerate amphotericin B.

## Amphotericin B

Intravenous (I/V) amphotericin B deoxycholate– More nephrotoxic, less costly

- dose is 1 to 1.5 mg/ kg daily

Intravenous (I/V) liposomal amphotericin B– less nephrotoxic, more costly

- dose is 5 mg/kg daily

**Prevention of nephrotoxicity amphotericin B**

use of sodium supplementation (example-intravenous saline) along with avoiding dehydration decreases the risk of nephrotoxicity associated with amphotericin B administration.

## Oral posaconazole

Oral posaconazole, delayed-release tablets (300 mg every 12 hours on the first day, 300 mg once daily) taken with food if possible.

## Oral isavuconazole

- Oral isavuconazole -Loading doses of 200 mg ( two capsules) of oral isavuconazole should be given every 8 hours for six doses, followed by 200 mg orally once daily starting 12 to 24 hours after the last loading dose.
- a wider spectrum of antifungal activity.
- excellent oral bioavailability not reliant on food intake or gastric pH
- available in an intravenous formulation, which does not contain the nephrotoxic solubilizing agent cyclodextrin.
- Switching between oral and IV forms does not require dose adjustment.

## Duration of the medical treatment -

- Successful courses of amphotericin B typically last 4-6 weeks.
- Primary or salvage isavuconazole or Posaconazole therapy may be continued for several months
- Therapy should continue until there is the clinical resolution of the signs and symptoms of infection, as well as resolution of radiographic signs of active disease.

*"Key to treatment is early and progressive surgical debridement of the necrosed tissue along with Intravenous antifungal therapy(amphotericin-b)"*

## Prognosis

- Mucormycosis has a fulminant fatal clinical pattern.
- The survival rates among patients with invasive sinus disease without cerebral involvement may be as high as 50-80%.
- If the infection spreads to the brain, the case fatality rate can exceed 80%.
- Death may occur within 2 weeks, if mucormycosis is not treated or is unsuccessfully treated.

## Prevention of mucormycosis

➢ Steroids and Interleukin 6 (IL-6) inhibitors (tocilizumab) increase the risk of secondary infections as they are immunosuppressive drugs.

## Steroids

• **Chinese Thoracic Society**

states that steroids should be used with caution in patients with hypoxaemia with COVID-19 and dose administration should be less than 0.5 mg per kg per day methylprednisolone or equivalent and for a shorter duration of less than seven days. Short-term use is safe except for temporary hyperglycaemia.

• **NIH (National Institute of Health, a part of the US Department of Health and Human Services) treatment guidelines panel**

1) Panel recommends using dexamethasone 6 mg per day for up to 10 days or until hospital discharge in hospitalised patients who

are on mechanical ventilation or requiring supplemental oxygen.

2) Panel recommends against using dexamethasone for the treatment of patients who do not require supplemental oxygen.

3) If dexamethasone is not available panel recommends alternatives such as prednisolone, methylprednisolone or hydrocortisone.

## WHO Practical issues for the use of systemic corticosteroids

• Medication route: orally or intravenously.

<u>Equivalent doses of steroids in COVID-19 for 7 to 10 days in patients requiring supplemental oxygen or mechanical ventilation</u>

- Dexamethasone- 6 mg once daily
- Methylprednisolone -32 mg (8 mg 6 hourly or 16 mg 12 hourly)
- Hydrocortisone –160 mg (50 mg 8 hourly or 100 mg 12 hourly)
- Prednisolone 40 mg once daily

**Use of Interleukin *6* (IL-6) inhibitor (tocilizumab) in selected patients with the following indications-**

The **NIH (National Institute of health) US Panel** recommends using tocilizumab (single intravenous [IV] dose of tocilizumab 8 mg/kg actual body weight up to 800 mg) in combination with dexamethasone (6 mg daily for up to 10 days) in certain hospitalized patients who are exhibiting rapid respiratory decompensation due to COVID-19. These patients are:-

- Recently hospitalized patients (i.e., within the first 3 days of admission) who have been admitted to the intensive care unit (ICU) within the prior 24 hours and who require invasive mechanical ventilation, non-invasive ventilation, or high-flow nasal cannula (HFNC) oxygen (>0.4 FiO2/30 L/min of oxygen flow)
- Recently hospitalized patients (i.e., within the first 3 days of admission) not admitted to the ICU who have rapidly increased oxygen needs and require non-invasive ventilation or HFNC

oxygen and who have significantly increased markers of inflammation (CRP ≥75 mg/L).

**Use of monoclonal antibodies in selected patients with the following indications-**

- o Monoclonal antibodies can block or reduce immune cells and cytokines and can lead to an increased risk of infection.
- o Should be used in patients with mild to moderate COVID-19 who do not require hospitalization or supplemental oxygen or who are at high risk of progression to severe disease.